NutriBullet Weight Loss Smoothies

All Under 200 Calories

- includes recipes, calorie content, nutritional information, & health benefits.

By Karen Simms

Copyright © 2015 by Karen Simms

All rights reserved; no part of this publication may be reproduced, stored in a retrieval system, or transmitted in any form or by any means, electronic, mechanical, photocopying, recording or otherwise without the prior written permission of the publisher.

Disclaimer

Before reading or following any of the recipes in this book, it is very important to familiarize yourself with the safety precautions outlined in Chapter 1. The author does not hold any responsibility or liability towards any person or entity regarding any loss or damage incurred, or alleged to have incurred, directly or indirectly, through the use of the information provided in this book.

As part of a healthy weight loss program, a health practitioner such as a dietician or GP should be consulted with regards to healthy weight loss. Those suffering from any nut allergies should avoid all recipes containing nuts or seeds.

This book is written to supplement the Nutribullet and is in no way affiliated with Nutribullet LLC. Nutribullet LLC was not involved in any of the recipe experimenting and developing, and is not affiliated with any of the recipes in this book.

First published March 2015

ISBN-13: 978-1508823605
ISBN-10: 150882360X

Introduction

1	Using the Nutribullet	9
2	Calorie Content of Smoothie Ingredients	13
3	Benefits of Smoothie Ingredients	23
4	How to Make the Perfect Weight Loss Smoothie	33
5	Weight Loss Smoothie Recipes Under 200 Calories	36

Berry Supreme — 36
Green Tea Sizzler — 37
Coconut Wonder — 38
Lime Delight — 39
Detox Blitz — 40
Weight Loss Wonder — 41
Cellulite Buster — 42
Berry Powerhouse — 43
Hearty Cocoa — 44
Citrus Burst — 45
Acai Sunrise — 46
Tropical Glory — 47
Zingy Lemon — 48
Slim Spinach — 49
Summer Sun — 50
Flax to the Max — 51
Spirulina Cleanser — 52
Cinnamon Sensation — 53
Pina Colada Treat — 54
Minty Fresh — 55

Precious Papaya	56
Hail to Kale	57
Pepper Pie	58
Orange Supreme	59
Green Delight	60
Magic Melon	61
Red River	62
Divine Nectarine	63
Gone Green	64
Glowing Green	65
Banana Glory	66
Secret Sesame	67
Skinny Minnie	68
Gracious Grapes	69
Liver Tonic	70
Veggie Heaven	71
Detox Deli	72
Vitamin Frenzy	73
Cleanse & Detox	74
Green Earth	75
Goji Crush	76
Ocean Spring	77
Passionate Green	78
Green Attack	79
Fruit Punch	80
Antioxidant Apple	81
Tangy Tank	82
Ginger Banana	83
Orange & Lime	84
Berry Star	85
Detox Splash	86
Summer Wave	87
Green Blast	88

Fruitilicious	89
Nutrient Ninja	90
Berry Rejuvenator	91
Leafy Green	92
Amazing Asparagus	93
The Green King	94
Orange Infusion	95
References	96

Introduction

If there is one thing that all nutritionists, dieticians, and dieters themselves agree on, it is that personal motivation is the key to weight loss success. How many times have we said to ourselves, "I don't have the time", or "It takes too long to prepare healthy meals", or "I'll be hungry all the time", or "I don't like healthy food." These excuses can often stop us in our tracks before we even start.

After these poor excuses, the next most common problem we face when dieting is boredom. This typically occurs when our initial motivation or enthusiasm for losing weight wears off, and we become fed up at watching what calories we are taking in, and worrying about what foods we can and cannot eat. We become dispirited, and this is when feelings of demotivation and disinterest start to take over. Unfortunately, poor excuses and boredom lead to the inevitable failure at losing weight successfully. Until now that is.

No more excuse for poor excuses!

Thankfully, our dieting prayers were answered not so long ago when the Nutribullet was introduced into our lives. All those excuses we once had were no more. No time? It takes 20 seconds to blend and 20 seconds to clean! It takes too long to prepare healthy meals? It should take you no more than 5 – 7 minutes to prepare the ingredients. I don't like healthy food? What is not to love about all the various recipes and concoctions you can come up with?! I'll be hungry all the time? Speaking from personal experience, this shouldn't be the case. If you include roughage in your Nutribullet smoothie such as sesame seeds, flax seeds, or almonds, you should feel full and satisfied.

Nutribullet sales have soared over the last couple of years, and continue to do so. John Lewis, a popular British retailer, reported selling 1 Nutribullet every 30 seconds on "Black Friday" in November 2014. The term "Nutribullet" has passed the lips of most health conscious people out there and it is fast becoming a staple in everyone's kitchen. It is not difficult to figure out why this is the case. I have made countless healthy smoothies using my Nutribullet. I have made pancakes (ok, not so healthy), homemade spaghetti Bolognese sauce, soups, bread mixes, and even homemade cleansers and creams for my face! This list is endless. And all recipes took seconds. It just doesn't get any better than that.

There has never been an easier way to introduce healthy, balanced, and wholesome weight loss smoothies into your life. Because the Nutribullet works by extracting ALL of the nutrients from the fruit and vegetables (including leafy greens) and breaking them down into their most digestive form, the digestive system is more capable of absorbing the essential vitamins, minerals, fiber, and phytonutrients from the food. This gives our body the kick start it needs to start burning fat cells at a healthy rate, boosting metabolism, regulating blood sugar levels, and increasing our energy levels.

The Nutribullet is an incredibly quick and efficient way of introducing all of the vital nutrients our body needs to function at its optimum level.

The recipes in this book have been designed with 2 things in mind:

1. A calorie content of under 200.

2. A recipe that includes ingredients to encourage HEALTHY weight loss.

While all the recipes are under 200 calories, I have provided the calorie content of all individual ingredients in a separate chapter, so you can come up with your own recipes if you wish. Chapter 2 will give you some useful tips on compiling your own weight loss recipe and advise on what ingredients not to use.

Whether you decide to substitute your breakfast for a healthy smoothie, or add one in as a healthy snack, always remember to have a balanced, wholesome diet and approach your weight loss program in a sensible manner. Your goal should be long term weight loss which is something that can easily be achieved by adding delicious, healthy Nutribullet smoothies to your diet.

1

Using the Nutribullet

The secret to the power of the Nutribullet is the 600/900-watt motor combined with the extractor blade and cyclonic action that pulverizes each ingredient, including the stem, pulp, seeds, peel, skin, and greens, extracting all possible nutrients from within the piece of fruit or vegetable. The Nutribullet:

- ✓ Shatters through stems.
- ✓ Smashes open seeds.
- ✓ Slices through tough skins.
- ✓ Chops up nuts with ease.

Using the Nutribullet is so quick and easy to use; it is as simple as A, B, C!

A – Load

B – Extract

C – Enjoy

For the purpose of this book, the measurements I have used are as follows:

1 cup = 250 mls or 9 fl oz
1/2 cup = 125 mls or 4.5 fl oz
1/3 cup = 80 mls or 3 fl oz
1/4 cup = 60 mls or 2.25 fl oz

Getting started

Step 1
If you are using leafy greens, such as mint leaves, parsley, spinach, or kale, add these first.

Step 2
Add any prepared fruit or vegetables including carrots, apples, peaches, celery, or cucumber.

Step 3
Add your smoothie boosts such as almonds, chia seeds, spirulina powder, or ground flax seeds.

Step 4
Pour in your liquid, which can be water (preferably filtered or distilled), coconut water, cooled teas, or fruit juices (be careful of the sugar content, particularly with weight loss smoothies). If you prefer a thinner smoothie, pour to the max line, however if you prefer a thicker smoothie, pour in less liquid. Never pour beyond the max line.

Note: if you prefer to mill your nuts or seeds before placing them into the cup, you can use the milling blade that comes with your Nutribullet. This turns dry ingredients into powders.

It is as simple as that! Now you are ready to experience the health and vitality that regular use of the Nutribullet can bring you, and when people start to comment on how radiant your skin looks or how trim your waist line is becoming, you can simply smile, and ask them if they have ever heard of the Nutribullet. If they haven't, then pay it forward. Enjoy!

Safety precautions when using the Nutribullet

- As soon as you get the product home, make sure you thoroughly read through the manufacturer's guidelines to familiarize yourself with how the product works, how it should be cleaned, and how to use it.

- As soon as you have finished making your smoothie, rinse the blades in warm (not hot) water to remove debris. If left to dry, the debris hardens and sticks to the blades, and can be a nightmare to remove. Do not put the blades into the dishwater.

- Likewise, as soon as you have finished with the cup, rinse in warm, soapy water (not hot) to remove debris. Dry immediately. The cups can be placed in the dishwasher but only on a normal cycle. And never soak in boiling water as this will damage the cups.

- When you are cleaning the Nutribullet itself, always make sure it is unplugged. Use a damp cloth only. Never submerge the Nutribullet in water and never place in the dishwater.

- Most definitely keep out of reach of children. Remember the Nutribullet is powerful.

- When the Nutribullet is plugged in, never put your hands or any utensils near the power base.

- Always place the Nutribullet on a hard surface such as your kitchen counter or table.

- ❖ Be careful with the lead and make sure it cannot be reached by children.

- ❖ It is not recommended to blend for more than 60 seconds at one time to prevent motor damage. Personally I find that 20 seconds is time enough to make the perfect blend.

- ❖ Do not put any part of the Nutribullet, including the cups, into the microwave or oven.

- ❖ Do not overfill the Nutribullet.

- ❖ Do not blend carbonated drinks as the build up of gas can lead to bursting of the container.

- ❖ Do not blend hot liquids of any description. **Green tea is an excellent choice of drink for a weight loss smoothie, and as such I have used the tea several times. Always allow the tea to cool and remove the tea bag before pouring into the Nutribullet cup.**

- ❖ Do not use the following seeds:

  - Plum pits
  - Peach pits
  - Cherry pits
  - Apricot pits
  - Apple seeds

2

Calorie Content of Smoothie Ingredients

Fruit Under 50 Calories

Cranberries – 1 cup, whole (100g):
Calories - 46
Dietary fiber - 4.6g
Sugar - 4g

Goji Berries – 1 tablespoon (0.625 oz):
Calories - 42
Dietary fiber -2.1g
Sugar - 6g

Kiwi Fruit - (2" dia) (69g):
Calories - 42
Dietary fiber - 2.1g
Sugar - 6g

Lemon - 1 wedge or slice (7g):
Calories - 2
Dietary fiber - 0.2g
Sugar – 0.2g

Lime - 1 fruit (2" dia) (67g):
Calories - 20
Dietary fiber - 1.9g
Sugar - 1.1g

Passion Fruit – 1 fruit without refuse (18g):
Calories - 17
Dietary fiber - 1.9g
Sugar - 2g

Plum -1 fruit (approx 2" dia) (66g):
Calories - 30
Dietary fiber - 0.9g
Sugar - 7g

Starfruit - 1 medium sized (approx 3.5" long) (91g):
Calories - 28
Dietary fiber - 2.5g
Sugar - 3.6g

Strawberries - 1 cup, halves (152g):
Calories - 49
Dietary fiber - 3g
Sugar - 7g

Tangerine - 1 medium sized (approx 2.5" dia) (88g):
Calories - 47
Dietary fiber - 1.6g
Sugar - 9g

Watermelon - 1 cup, diced (152g):
Calories - 46
Dietary fiber - 0.6g
Sugar - 9g

Fruit from 51 to 100 Calories

Apple - 1 medium sized (3" dia) (182g):
Calories - 95
Dietary fiber - 4.4g
Sugar - 19g

Blackberries – 1 cup (144g):
Calories - 62
Dietary fiber - 8g
Sugar - 7g

Blueberries – 1 cup (148g):
Calories - 85
Dietary fiber - 3.6g
Sugar - 15g

Cantaloupe - 1 cup, diced (156g):
Calories - 53
Dietary fiber – 1.4g
Sugar - 12g

Cherries, sweet - 1 cup, without pits (154g):
Calories - 97
Dietary fiber - 3.2g
Sugar - 20g

Grapefruit, pink, red, and white - ½ fruit (approx 3.75" dia) (123g):
Calories - 52
Dietary fiber - 2g
Sugar - 8g

Mango - 1 cup of pieces (165g):
Calories - 99
Dietary fiber - 2.6g
Sugar - 23g

Nectarine - 1 medium sized (approx 2.5" dia) (142g):
Calories - 62
Dietary fiber - 2.4g
Sugar - 11g

Orange - 1 medium sized (approx 2.5" dia) (131g):
Calories - 62
Dietary fiber - 3.1g
Sugar - 12g

Papaya - 1 small sized (157g):
Calories - 67
Dietary fiber - 2.7g
Sugar - 12g

Peach - 1 medium sized (approx 2" dia) (150g):
Calories - 59
Dietary fiber - 2.2g
Sugar - 13g

Pineapple -1 cup of chunks (165g):
Calories - 82
Dietary fiber - 2.3g
Sugar - 16g

Raspberries - 1 cup (123g):
Calories - 65
Dietary fiber - 8g
Sugar - 5g

Fruit Over 100 Calories

Avocado - 1 medium sized (201g):
Calories - 322
Dietary fiber - 14g
Sugar - 1.3g

Banana - 1 medium sized (approx 7" long) (118g):
Calories - 105
Dietary fiber - 3.1g
Sugar - 14g

Grapes - 1 cup (151g):
Calories - 104
Dietary fiber - 1g
Sugar - 23g

Pear - 1 medium sized (178g):
Calories - 102
Dietary fiber - 6g
Sugar - 17g

Vegetables/Leafy Greens Under 50 Calories

Arugula/Salad Rocket - 1 cup (20g):
Calories - 6
Dietary fiber - 0.2g
Sugar - 0.2g

Asparagus - 1 cup (134g):
Calories - 27
Dietary fiber - 2.8g
Sugar - 2.5g

Beets - 1 beet (2" dia) (82g):
Calories - 35
Dietary fiber - 2.3g
Sugar - 6g

Bok Choy/Pak Choy – 1 cup, shredded (70g):
Calories - 9
Dietary fiber - 0.7g
Sugar - 0.8g

Broccoli - 1 spear (about 5" long) (31g):
Calories - 11
Dietary fiber - 0.8g
Sugar - 0.5g

Cabbage - 1 cup, chopped (89g):
Calories - 22
Dietary fiber - 2.2g
Sugar - 2.8g

Carrot - 1 medium sized (61g):
Calories - 25
Dietary fiber - 1.7g
Sugar - 2.9g

Cauliflower - 1 floweret (13g):
Calories - 3
Dietary fiber - 0.3g
Sugar - 0.2g

Celery - 1 stalk, medium (approx 7.5" long) (40g):
Calories - 6
Dietary fiber - 0.6g
Sugar - 0.7g

Collard Greens – 1 cup, chopped (36g):
Calories - 11
Dietary fiber - 1.4g
Sugar - 0.2g

Cucumber - 1 medium sized, with peel (approx 8" long) (301g):
Calories - 47
Dietary fiber - 1.5g
Sugar - 5g

Green Bell Pepper - 1 medium sized (approx 2" dia) (119g):
Calories - 24
Dietary fiber - 2g
Sugar - 2.9g

Kale - 1 cup, chopped (67g):
Calories - 33
Dietary fiber - 1g
Sugar - 0g

Mint Leaves – 2 leaves (0g):
Calories - 0
Dietary fiber - 0g
Sugar - 0g

Parsley - 1 cup, chopped (60g):
Calories - 22
Dietary fiber - 2g
Sugar - 0.5g

Red Pepper, Sweet – 1 medium sized (approx 2.5" dia) (119g):
Calories - 37
Dietary fiber - 2g
Sugar - 5g

Romaine Lettuce – 1 cup, shredded (47g):
Calories - 8
Dietary fiber - 1g
Sugar - 0.6g

Spinach - 1 cup (30g):
Calories -7
Dietary fiber - 0.7g
Sugar - 0.1g

Swiss chard - 1 cup (36g):
Calories - 7
Dietary fiber - 0.6g
Sugar - 0.4g

Tomato, red - 1 medium whole (approx 2" dia) (123g):
Calories - 22
Dietary fiber - 1.5g
Sugar - 3.2g

Watercress - 1 cup, chopped (34g):
Calories - 4
Dietary fiber - 0.2g
Sugar - 0.1g

Zucchini - 1 medium sized (196g):
Calories - 33
Dietary fiber - 2g
Sugar - 4.9g

Smoothie Boosters Under 50 Calories

Almonds - 1 almond (1.2g):
Calories - 7
Dietary fiber - 0.1g
Sugar - 0g

Cinnamon - 1 teaspoon (2.6g):
Calories - 6
Dietary fiber - 1.4g
Sugar - 0.1g

Coconut Water – 1 serving 250ml, (Brand: Vita Coco):
Calories - 45
Dietary fiber - 1g
Sugar - 12.5g

Flax Seeds - 1 tablespoon ground flax seed (7g):
Calories - 37
Dietary fiber - 1.9g
Sugar - 0.1g

Ginger - 5 slices (1" dia) (11g):
Calories - 9
Dietary fiber - 0.2g
Sugar - 0.2g

Green Tea – 1 cup, 250ml:
Calories - 2
Dietary fiber - 0g
Sugar - 0g

Matcha Green Tea Powder - 1 teaspoon (4.7g)
Calories - 14.9
Dietary fiber - 1.5g
Sugar - 0g

Spirulina - 1 level tablespoon (7g)
Calories - 20
Dietary fiber - 0g
Sugar - 0g

Turmeric - 1 teaspoon (2.2g):
Calories - 8
Dietary fiber - 0.5g
Sugar - 0.1g

Smoothie Boosters from 51 to 100 Calories

Chia Seeds - 1 tablespoon (13g):
Calories - 60
Dietary fiber - 6g
Sugar - 0g

Pumpkin Seeds - 1 tablespoon (15g):
Calories - 56
Dietary fiber - 0.6g
Sugar - 0g

Sesame Seeds - 1 tablespoon (9g):
Calories - 52
Dietary fiber - 1.1g
Sugar - 0g

3

Benefits of Smoothie Ingredients

<u>Fruit</u>

Apples – very low in saturated fat and cholesterol with an impressive 4 grams of soluble fiber, an apple makes for a filling, satisfying snack. They are also a great source of vitamin C, calcium, phosphorus, potassium, and magnesium.

Avocados – while avocados contain monounsaturated fat which is very beneficial to our health, helping to lower cholesterol, they have a high calorie content and should therefore be used sparingly in a weight loss smoothie. Phytonutrients, vitamins C & K, potassium, and dietary fiber are also present in this healthy treat.

Bananas – the dietary fiber found in bananas not only enhances a weight loss program but it also helps to reduce the risk of heart disease, and promotes regular bowel movement. Vitamin B6, vitamin C, and potassium are also found in abundance in bananas.

Blackberries – rich in vitamins, minerals, and antioxidants, blackberries pack a powerful nutritious punch as well as being low in calories. Their high fiber content helps to boost metabolism, eliminate cravings, and burn more calories.

Blueberries – regarded by many as having the highest level of antioxidants among all fruits and vegetables, blueberries are excellent at preventing damage to our cell structure and DNA, they promote healthy, strong connective tissue, and improve blood sugar and insulin levels. Vitamins A, C, and E, selenium, iron, and zinc are also present.

Cherries – cherries are loaded with anti-inflammatory and anti-aging properties, they are high in soluble fiber, low in calories, and are a perfect choice for satisfying your sweet cravings. Along with their superior antioxidant content, they are an excellent source of vitamins A and C, potassium, zinc, and iron.

Cranberries – packed with flavonoids and polyphenols, cranberries help to protect against cancer, reduce the risk of heart disease, treat urinary tract infections, and prevent the formation of kidney stones. Cranberries are an excellent choice for a weight loss smoothie due to their high fiber content, low sugar content, and low calorie content (46 calories for 1 cup, whole).

Goji Berries – these beautiful berries demonstrate strong antioxidant properties with immune boosting results. They are also known to have a positive effect on insulin resistance. They are a rich source of carotenoids and vitamin C, while possessing a high fiber content.

Grapefruit – a staple in any weight loss plan, grapefruit helps to reduce fatty tissue, regulate blood sugar levels, and lower bad cholesterol. They are loaded with vitamins A, C, B1, and B5.

Grapes – grapes, particularly red skin grapes, contain a substance called resveratrol that has magical anti-aging effects on the skin. They are loaded with antioxidants and potassium which help to promote a healthy heart and significantly reduce bad cholesterol.

Kiwi – a wonderful source of vitamin C, kiwi fruit's many benefits include anti-aging, anti-inflammatory, protection against free radical damage, regulation of blood sugar levels, and strengthening of the immune system. It is also an excellent source of dietary fiber and potassium.

Lemon – lemons contain effective detoxification properties, helping to cleanse the liver of toxins. As a result, weight loss is accelerated, the appearance of cellulite is reduced, skin health is improved, and our energy increases. Lemons are also another wonderful source of vitamin C.

Lime – limes are packed with flavor and nutritional benefits including protection against bacterial and viral infections, skin care, and protection against free radical damage. Limes are very low in saturated fat and cholesterol, they are an excellent source of vitamin C, and have a high fiber content.

Mango – mangos are nutritionally rich, containing high levels of vitamin A and beta carotene. They are a perfect choice for promoting digestive health due to their high fiber content, and make a great addition to a weight loss smoothie.

Nectarine – similar to peaches, nectarines are a great snack when on a weight loss program as they contain only 63 calories for one medium sized fruit. They are also fat free and are an excellent source of fiber and potassium.

Orange – oranges contain an abundance of antioxidants, antiviral, anti-inflammatory, anti-aging, antifungal, and antibacterial properties. They help to lower bad cholesterol, combat cancer, fight infection, and help to reduce the risk of cardiovascular disease. The pulp is an excellent source of fiber so don't forget to add it all into your smoothie.

Papaya – the weight loss benefits of papaya fruit are endless. It is one of the best sources of digestive enzymes, helping to promote the proper digestion of food. It has a high fiber content which helps to promote weight loss by creating a feeling of fullness, and its calcium, potassium, and vitamin C content help to boost our metabolism and break down fat cells.

Passion Fruit – this fruit is a good source of dietary fiber, is low in calories, and is a rich source of antioxidants, minerals, and vitamins. Passion fruit seeds are also an excellent source of nutrients and should therefore be added to your smoothie. Healthy skin, cell growth, good vision, and your immune system all benefit from eating this delicious fruit.

Peaches – their low calorie content and low glycemic load make peaches a beneficial fruit to help regulate blood sugar levels. They also contain valuable anti-inflammatory and anti-cancer properties.

Pears – compared to most other fruit on our list, 1 medium sized pear contains 102 calories per serving, which means it should be used sparingly in weight loss smoothies, particularly those under 200 calories. That aside, pears contain a wealth of healthy nutrients including vitamins C, K, B2 and B3.

Pineapple – a pineapple's low fat and calorie content, together with its fiber-rich content make is an excellent choice for a healthy weight loss smoothie. It is rich in a enzyme called bromelain which helps to improve the body's digestive process and reduce inflammation.

Plum – with high levels of potassium, plums help to reduce high blood pressure and reduce the risk of stroke. Plums are also low in calories (30 calories for one 2" dia fruit) and contain no saturated fat. Their fiber and antioxidant properties help to regulate the smooth running of the digestive system.

Raspberries – raspberries are nutrient rich and packed full of antioxidants. They contain excellent anti-inflammatory and antioxidant properties helping to protect us from obesity, cancer, heart disease, and constipation. They are one of the highest fiber-rich fruits on the planet, and this, together with their low calorie content, make them a valuable addition to any weight loss smoothie.

Starfruit – starfruit is an excellent source of vitamins A and C, and fiber, which helps to boost our metabolism, fight against infection, promote healthy bowel movements, and lower bad cholesterol. It is low in calories and also contains low levels of fat.

Strawberries – little nutrient powerhouses, strawberries contain vitamin C, dietary fiber, potassium, magnesium, and folate in abundance. They are an excellent choice for a weight loss smoothie due to their low calorie content, plus they taste delicious.

Tangerine – tangerines are a valuable source of fiber and flavonoids, and are also a rich source of vitamin C. They contain an array of health benefits including helping to eliminate toxins from the body, preventing cholesterol build up in the gut, increasing energy levels, and promoting wound healing.

Watermelon – watermelons are a popular food choice for dieters due to their filling effect. This is due to their high water content (approximately 95%). They are also a rich source of vitamins A and C, along with lycopene, potassium, and magnesium.

Vegetables/Leafy Greens

Arugula/Salad Rocket – a strong tasting, peppery leaf, arugula (also known as rocket) contains large amounts of vitamin K and calcium, both vital for healthy gums and bones. It also has high levels of chlorophyll which is an important nutrient for detoxification of the liver.

Asparagus – asparagus is an excellent source of potassium and fiber, essential for promoting good digestive health. It is low in calories and high is vitamins A, B, and K. It also contains a healthy dose of flavonoids, helping to protect against cancer.

Beets – this nutritious root vegetable is a valuable tonic for the liver as it helps to purify and cleanse the blood. Beets are loaded with potassium and are a good source of folate, helping to reduce the risk of heart disease and promote healthy blood vessels.

Bok Choy/Pak Choy – a mild tasting Chinese cabbage, bok choy packs a punch when it comes to its calcium and potassium content. It also contains all the essential vitamins and minerals needed to keep a body healthy and strong. The nutritional benefits of boy choy along with its low calorie content make it an ideal choice for a healthy weight loss smoothie.

Broccoli – a nutritional wonder food, beloved broccoli contains an abundance of nutrients including protein, vitamin C, potassium, fiber, vitamin A, folate, magnesium, phosphorus, beta-carotene, and cancer-fighting antioxidants. It is a mild tasting root vegetable in a smoothie.

Cabbage – both red and green cabbage provides a highly concentrated source of vitamin C, fiber, calcium, iodine, and beta-carotene. It is a mild tasting leafy green which helps to lower bad cholesterol, fight inflammation, and promote strong and healthy connective tissue.

Carrots – packed full of antioxidants, carrots possess powerful cancer-fighting properties, as well as valuable eye health benefits. They are rich in fiber and have excellent detoxification capabilities.

Cauliflower – cauliflower is very low in calories but high in fiber, potassium, and vitamin C. It is excellent at helping to eliminate a build up of toxins from the liver, and is an important source of dietary fiber for digestive health.

Celery – a popular choice for a weight loss smoothie, celery acts as a powerful appetite controller, helping to curb carb cravings in between meals. When added to a smoothie, it helps to fill you up as well as promoting healthy digestion.

Collard Greens – a strong tasting leafy green, collard greens are jam packed full of calcium, potassium, magnesium, and fiber. They are also an excellent source of vitamins A and K. Collard greens are effective at helping to reduce bad cholesterol levels, keeping our heart healthy and strong.

Cucumber – a powerful diuretic, cucumber helps to rehydrate the body, keeping the skin and cells healthy. Due to its low calorie and high water content, cucumber is an ideal addition to a weight loss smoothie as it helps rid the body of harmful toxins, promotes healthy digestion, and regulates bowel movements.

Kale – a mild tasting leafy green, kale is a nutrient powerhouse, loaded with antioxidants, vitamins A, C, and K, omega 3 fatty acids, calcium, iron, and essential dietary fiber. It is a valuable source of protein, and contains a valuable supply of beta-carotene. A popular choice in a weight loss smoothie, this is one leafy green that should not be overlooked.

Pepper, Green & Red (Sweet) – naturally low in calories, peppers are an excellent source of vitamins A and C. They also contain a good amount of vitamin K, vital for healthy blood clotting, bone health, and preventing heart disease. They contain plenty of vitamin C which helps to keep the immune system strong and prevents premature aging.

Mint Leaves – with a spicy taste, mint leaves contain potent antioxidants to give any smoothie a healthy boost. They are excellent at preventing and treating certain allergies, and promoting digestion by stimulating efficient bile flow.

Parsley – parsley is a strong tasting leafy green, rich in many vital vitamins and minerals including vitamins A, B12, C, and K, folate, iron, and potassium. It helps to reduce fluid retention, reduces the risk of heart disease, and promotes healthy bones and joints.

Romaine Lettuce – romaine lettuce contains a rich supply of vitamin C (1 head contains more vitamin C than an orange!), calcium, iron, beta carotene, and protein. It has a high water content and low calorie content, making it a popular choice for a weight loss smoothie.

Spinach – spinach is one of the richest sources of nutrients on the planet. It provides the body with healthy amounts of fiber, calcium, phosphorus, selenium, and vitamins C, E and K. It works wonders for our energy levels, enhances skin complexion, promotes strong connective tissue, and boosts our immune system. A mild tasting leafy green, spinach is an excellent addition to any smoothie.

Swiss chard – a mild tasting leafy green, chard provides many of the nutrients our body needs to stay healthy and strong including beta-carotene, zinc, lutein, and vitamins A, C and E. It's valuable fiber content helps to regulate weight loss by promoting a healthy digestive system.

Tomatoes – technically a fruit, tomatoes are classified as a vegetable because they are generally used as such. Regardless of their status, tomatoes provide a rich source of cancer-fighting lycopene as well as powerful phytochemicals and vitamin C.

Watercress – a fantastic addition to a weight loss smoothie due to its ridiculously low calorie content, watercress packs a nutritious punch. Calcium, magnesium, vitamin C, iron, vitamin A, and vitamin K are just some of the essential nutrients contained in this miracle superfood.

Zucchini – ideal for weight loss due to its low calorie content, lack of fat and cholesterol, and high fiber content, a zucchini (also known as a courgette) provides a good source of potassium, vitamin A and C, and various antioxidants such as carotenes and lutein.

Smoothie Boosters

Almonds – these tasty nuts are packed with essential vitamins, minerals, protein, and fiber. They act as a wonderful tonic for the heart, reducing the risk of heart disease, lowering bad cholesterol, protecting the artery walls from damage, and helping to lower high blood pressure.

Chia Seeds – chia seeds are high in protein, fiber, and antioxidants. The high fiber content allows for slow absorption of food and therefore makes you feel fuller for longer. Chia seeds also lower the risk of type 2 diabetes.

Cinnamon – cinnamon contains high levels of antioxidants and antimicrobial properties. Its powerful health benefits range from protection from heart disease, blood sugar regulation, improvement in brain function, and protection against inflammation.

Coconut Water – coconut water is a perfect low-fat health drink which is cholesterol free, low in carbohydrates, packed with essential minerals, and loaded with B group vitamins. It helps to rehydrate the body, prevent premature aging, and regulate blood pressure and blood sugar levels.

Ginger – ginger is great for the digestive system, helping to promote the elimination of excessive gas, soothe intestinal problems, reduce the symptoms of nausea and vomiting, and prevent inflammation of the intestines.

Green Tea – loaded with antioxidants and nutrients, green tea has a powerful effect on the body, particularly when it comes to weight loss. It helps to speed up the burning of fat cells and can actually boost the metabolism. It also help to reduce the risk of cancer, lower heart disease, and delay the signs of aging.

Flax Seeds – flax seeds are an omega 3 powerhouse, and help to promote brain function, alleviate mood swings, improve joint health, and help to reduce the risk of bad cholesterol. They are also fiber-rich making them an ideal addition to a weight loss smoothie.

Matcha Green Tea Powder – matcha is a very concentrated form of green tea and contains super doses of chlorophyll, amino acids, flavonoids, and antioxidants. It holds an array of health benefits including improved concentration and protection from damaging free radicals.

Pumpkin Seeds – pumpkin seeds are a fantastic source of essential minerals such as selenium, zinc, magnesium, phosphorus, and potassium. They help to stabilize blood sugar levels, ensure a good night's sleep, and promote prostate health in men.

Sesame Seeds – this little seeds are made up of essential fatty acids, antioxidants, and vitamins. They help to strengthen cell development, reduce cholesterol, and build strong bones.

Spirulina – spirulina contains a wealth of nutrients including gamma linolenic acid (GLA), omega 3 fatty acids, various antioxidants, and essential vitamins and minerals. It helps to reduce high blood pressure, improve memory loss, reduce inflammation, and fight chronic disease.

Turmeric – turmeric acts as a powerful anti-inflammatory agent and helps to protect the body's cells against free radical damage from toxic food. It helps to alleviate the symptoms of depression and Alzheimer's disease, and reduces the risk of heart disease.

4

How to Make the Perfect Weight Loss Smoothie

Including smoothies as part of your healthy weight loss program could not be easier. Not only are they packed full of nutritious goodies such as vitamins, minerals, antioxidants, amino acids, healthy fats, fiber, and healthy enzymes, but thanks to the Nutribullet, they have become quick and simple to make.

However, when embarking on your weight loss program you should be aware that there are certain ingredients that should not be included in your smoothie, as they can really increase the calorie content possibly making the smoothie too fattening.

<u>Tips on how to make the perfect weight loss smoothie:</u>

- If you are adding a high calorie fruit such as grapes or a pear, always include a lower calorie fruit such as 1 cup of strawberry halves, or a kiwi. Adding vegetables, particularly leafy greens, will also bring down the calorie content. *Refer to chapter 2 for a calorie breakdown of individual fruit and vegetables.*

- Cow's milk and yogurt should be avoided as they can actually have the opposite effect and lead to obesity if used on a regular basis and in high amounts. The majority of healthy smoothies will contain calcium (especially if you use dark leafy greens such as kale, spinach, or cabbage) so you should not be losing out.

- Most vegetables are very low in calories, making 100% vegetable smoothies a great choice for weight loss. If you find the taste too bitter, simply add 2 – 3 wedges of lemon or 1 lime, to counteract the bitterness.

- Most protein powders contain high amounts of sugar (often up to 75g per serving, depending on the brand) and should therefore be avoided when making a weight loss smoothie. You can easily substitute protein powder for a serving of healthy flax seeds, spirulina, or pumpkin seeds.

- Fruit juices should be avoided as these are also high in sugar. Some natural juices can contain up to as much as 14 teaspoons of sugar which would be detrimental to your weight loss program. Filtered water or green tea are ideal choices. Coconut water is also a great substitute but bear in mind 250ml contains 45 calories so add ingredients accordingly.

- Avoid canned fruits or vegetables as these often contain added preservatives or sweeteners which lead to an increase in calories. Fresh produce is best, followed by frozen produce.

- While avocados are a nutritious addition to any smoothie, they are very high in calories so should be used with caution.

Having the correct information makes a world of a difference when making a healthy, low calorie weight loss smoothie. Avoid the ingredients listed in this chapter and follow the calorie counting in chapter 2, you cannot go wrong.

5

Weight Loss Smoothie Recipes

Berry Supreme

1 cup of spinach
1 cup of raspberries
1 cup of strawberry halves
½ cup of blackberries
1 tablespoon ground flax seeds
Filtered water

Directions:
Add the spinach followed by the berries, flax seed, and water. Blend until smooth.

Health Benefits:
- ❖ Helps prevent heart disease.
- ❖ Boosts the immune system.
- ❖ Reduces the risk of cancer.
- ❖ Protects against cell damage.
- ❖ Anti aging.

Nutritional Information

Calories: 189   Dietary Fiber: 17.6g   Protein: 5.7g   Fat: 4.7g   Sugar: 15.7g

Green Tea Sizzler

2 cups of collard greens
1 tablespoon of goji berries
2 lemon wedges, peeled
1 cup of cranberries
1 peach, cored
1 cup of cooled green tea

Directions:
Place the greens in the cup, followed by the fruit and goji berries. Pour in the cooled green tea. Top up with filtered water if necessary. Blend until smooth.

Health Benefits
- ❖ Excellent for helping with weight loss.
- ❖ Protects the liver from damage.
- ❖ Helps lower bad cholesterol.
- ❖ Anti-inflammatory.
- ❖ Regulates blood sugar levels.

Nutritional Information

Calories: 175   Dietary Fiber: 12.1g   Protein: 6.2g   Fat: 1g   Sugar: 23.8g

Coconut Wonder

1 cup of coconut water
1 cup of spring greens
1 cup of diced watermelon
4 broccoli spears
1 kiwi fruit, peeled

Directions:
Add the spring greens to the cup, followed by the fruit and broccoli. Add the coconut water and top up with filtered water if necessary. Blend until smooth.

Health Benefits
- Helps with healthy digestive function.
- Boosts hydration.
- Helps reduce blood pressure.
- Maintains smooth and healthy skin.
- Increases energy levels.

Nutritional Information

Calories: 185   Dietary Fiber: 6.9g   Protein: 5.3g   Fat: 1g   Sugar: 29.5g

Lime Delight

2 cups of spinach
½ cup of chopped parsley
1 carrot, peeled and sliced
1 celery stalk, sliced
1 lime, peeled
1 apple, cored
Filtered water

Directions:
Place the spinach into the cup, followed by the parsley, and remaining ingredients. Add the filtered water and blend until smooth.

Health Benefits
- Enhances mood.
- Decreases the risk of heart disease.
- Improves sleeping patterns.
- Helps to reduce fluid retention.
- Balances the blood's pH.

Nutritional Information

Calories: 171   Dietary Fiber: 11g   Protein: 3.7g   Fat: 1.2g   Sugar: 24.2g

Detox Blitz

½ cucumber, sliced
1 cup of strawberry halves
1 medium beet, peeled and chopped
1 cup of pineapple chunks
Filtered water

Directions:
Place all ingredients into the cup followed by the filtered water. Blend until smooth.

Health Benefits
- Improves circulation of blood.
- Boosts the immune system.
- Stimulates the digestive system.
- Excellent for bone health.
- Helps to improve memory and concentration.

Nutritional Information

Calories: 190   Dietary Fiber: 8.4g   Protein: 4.2g   Fat: 0.9g   Sugar: 31.5g

Weight Loss Wonder

1 cup of chopped kale
1 cup of spinach
1 celery stalk, sliced
2 lemon wedges, peeled
½ cucumber
1 cup of green tea
14 almonds

Directions:
Place the leafy greens into the cup followed by the remaining ingredients. Add the cooled green tea and top up with filtered water if necessary. Blend until smooth.

Health Benefits
- Flushes toxins from the liver.
- Increases the burning of fat cells.
- Improves brain function.
- Lowers the risk of cancer.
- Helps to lower bad cholesterol.

Nutritional Information

Calories: 174   Dietary Fiber: 4.9g   Protein: 5g   Fat: 14.9g   Sugar: 3.7g

Cellulite Buster

½ grapefruit, peeled
1 cup of dark green cabbage
4 broccoli spears
4 cauliflower flowerets
1 small papaya, cored
Filtered water

Directions:
Place the cabbage into the cup followed by the broccoli, cauliflower, and fruit. Add the filtered water to the max line and blend until smooth.

Health Benefits
- ❖ Helps to eliminate toxins from the body.
- ❖ Reduces the build up of fluid retention.
- ❖ Boosts metabolism.
- ❖ Promotes gum health.
- ❖ Supports the immune system.

Nutritional Information

Calories: 197   **Dietary Fiber:** 11.3g   **Protein:** 8.1g   **Fat:** 1.1g   **Sugar:** 25.6g

Berry Powerhouse

1 cup of blackberries
1 cup of raspberries
1 cup of strawberry halves
1 cup of green tea
1 level tablespoon of spirulina

Directions:
Place all the berries into the cup followed by the spirulina and cooled green tea. Top up with some filtered water if necessary. Blend until smooth.

Health Benefits
- Helps to reduce the absorption of fats.
- Burns calories faster.
- Clears toxins from the body.
- Helps to relieve indigestion.
- Promotes healthy skin and hair.

Nutritional Information

Calories: 198   Dietary Fiber: 19g   Protein: 8.5g   Fat: 3g   Sugar: 19g

Hearty Cocoa

1 cup of spinach
1 teaspoon of unsweetened cocoa powder
1 cup of strawberry halves
1 medium banana
½ cup of diced watermelon
Filtered water

Directions:
Place the spinach and fruit into the cup. Sprinkle in the cocoa powder and add the filtered water to the max line. Blend until smooth.

Health Benefits
- Maintains the production and development of cell.
- Helps to alleviate feelings of depression.
- Improves blood flow and helps lower blood pressure.
- Helps to reduce inflammation.
- Reduces the risk of heart disease.

Nutritional Information

Calories: 196   Dietary Fiber: 9.1g   Protein: 4.7g   Fat: 1.8g   Sugar: 25.6g

Citrus Burst

1 orange, peeled and cut into segments
1 lime, peeled and cut into segments
9 almonds
½ grapefruit, peeled
½ cup of crushed ice
Filtered water

Directions:

Place the fruit into the cup followed by the nuts, ice, and filtered water. Blend until smooth.

Health Benefits
- Helps in the treatment of stress.
- Helps to inhibit the growth of cancer cells.
- Protects the body from damaging free radicals.
- Accelerates wound healing.
- Anti-aging.

Nutritional Information

Calories: 197   Dietary Fiber: 7.9g   Protein: 4.5g   Fat: 5g   Sugar: 21.1g

Acai Sunrise

1 tablespoon of acai berries
1 cup of Swiss chard
1 beet, peeled and sliced
1 plum, cored
1 kiwi, peeled
1 tablespoon of sesame seeds
Filtered water

Directions:
Place the Swiss chard into the cut first followed by the fruit, acai berries, and sesame seeds. Add the filtered water and blend until smooth.

Health Benefits
- ❖ Helps to break down fat cells.
- ❖ Improves bone health.
- ❖ Improves muscle oxygenation during exercise.
- ❖ Boosts brain function.
- ❖ Helps to prevent iron deficiency.

Nutritional Information

Calories: 181   Dietary Fiber: 9g   Protein: 4.9g   Fat: 5.3g   Sugar: 21.4g

Tropical Glory

1 cup of romaine lettuce
1 cup of spinach
1 cup of pineapple chunks
1 cup of strawberry halves
1 cup of diced watermelon
1 cup of green tea

Directions:
Add the greens to the cup followed by the fruit. Pour in the cooled green tea and top up with filtered water if necessary. Blend until smooth.

Health Benefits
- Promotes healthy digestion.
- Anti-inflammatory.
- Boosts collagen synthesis, helping to keep the skin younger looking.
- Healthy hair and nails.
- Helps to strengthen the gums.

Nutritional Information

Calories: 194   Dietary Fiber: 7.6g   Protein: 4.3g   Fat: 1.1g   Sugar: 32.7g

Zingy Lemon

1 cup of watercress
2 celery stalks, sliced
½ cucumber, sliced
3 lemon wedges, peeled
1 cup of coconut water
1" piece of ginger, peeled

Directions:
Add the watercress to the cup followed by the celery, cucumber, lemon, and ginger. Pour in the coconut water and top up with filtered water if necessary. Blend until smooth.

Health Benefits
- Promotes cardiovascular health.
- Helps to relieve migraines.
- Works at relieving insomnia.
- Boosts energy levels.
- Increases metabolism of fats.

Nutritional Information

Calories: 100   Dietary Fiber: 4g   Protein: 2.9g   Fat: 0.5g   Sugar: 4.8g

Slim Spinach

2 cups of spinach
1 cup of chopped asparagus
3 broccoli spears
1 teaspoon of turmeric
1 cup of blueberries
1 cup of chopped kale
Filtered water

Directions:

Place the leafy green into the cup first followed by the broccoli, asparagus, and blueberries. Sprinkle the turmeric on top and finish off by adding filtered water. Blend until smooth.

Health Benefits
- Helps to combat chronic inflammation.
- Reduces oxidative damage to the cells.
- Helps to reduce feelings of depression.
- Lowers the risk of heart disease.
- Delays the sign of aging.

Nutritional Information

Calories: 170   Dietary Fiber: 11.7g   Protein: 11.7g   Fat: 3g   Sugar: 19.3g

Summer Sun

1 pear, cored
1 lime, peeled
1 cup of watermelon chunks
½ cup of blackberries
Filtered water
½ cup of crushed ice

Directions:
Add all of the fruit to the cup followed by the crushed ice and filtered water. Blend until smooth.

Health Benefits
- ❖ Helps to detoxify the liver and blood.
- ❖ Regulates blood pressure.
- ❖ Improves blood circulation.
- ❖ Strengthens the immune system.
- ❖ Helps to keep the body hydrated.

Nutritional Information

Calories: 199 Dietary Fiber: 12.5g Protein: 3g Fat: 0.9g Sugar: 30.6g

Flax to the Max

1 cup of whole cranberries
2 carrots, peeled and sliced
4 cauliflower flowerets
1 cup of spinach
1 tablespoon of ground flax seeds
1 cup of green tea

Directions:
Place the spinach into the cup followed by the cranberries, carrots, cauliflower, and flax seeds. Top up the ingredients with the cooled green tea and blend until smooth.

Health Benefits
- ❖ Lowers the risk of diabetes, cancer, and heart disease.
- ❖ Regulates blood glucose levels.
- ❖ Keeps the heart healthy.
- ❖ Encourages strong, healthy hair.
- ❖ Eye health.

Nutritional Information

Calories: 154 Dietary Fiber: 11.8g Protein: 4.6g Fat: 3.6g Sugar: 6.4g

Spirulina Cleanser

1 peach, cored
1 cup of chopped kale
1 cup of raspberries
1 level tablespoon of spirulina
1 cup of green tea

Directions:
Add the leafy greens to the cup followed by the fruit. Sprinkle the spirulina on the top and pour in the cooled green tea. Top up with filtered water if necessary and blend until smooth.

Health Benefits
- Helps to remove toxins from the liver and blood.
- Speeds up the body's metabolism.
- Boosts the body's intake of iron.
- Helpful in treating allergic reactions.
- Increases the burning of fat cells during exercise.

Nutritional Information

Calories: 179   Dietary Fiber: 11.2g   Protein: 9.8g   Fat: 2.8g   Sugar: 18g

Cinnamon Sensation

1 nectarine, cored
1 medium banana, peeled and sliced
1 cup of spinach
½ teaspoon of cinnamon
Filtered water

Directions:
Place the spinach into the cup followed by the nectarine and banana. Sprinkle the cinnamon on top and add the filtered water. Blend until smooth.

Health Benefits
- ❖ Increases energy levels.
- ❖ Improves skin tone and elasticity.
- ❖ Protects against viral and bacterial infections.
- ❖ Helps to reduce fluid retention.
- ❖ Promotes regular bowel movement.

Nutritional Information

Calories: 177   Dietary Fiber: 7.6g   Protein: 4.3g   Fat: 0.7g   Sugar: 25.1g

Pina Colada Treat

1 cup of pineapple chunks
½ cup of whole cranberries
½ cup of diced cantaloupe
1 cup of coconut water
½ cup of crushed ice

Directions:
Place all of the fruit in the cup followed by the ice cubes and coconut milk. Blend until smooth.

Health Benefits
- ❖ Helps to maintain the elasticity of blood vessels.
- ❖ Protects against harmful free radicals.
- ❖ Helps to improve the health of the digestive system.
- ❖ Regulates blood sugar levels.
- ❖ Cleanses the liver of toxins.

Nutritional Information

Calories: 199   Dietary Fiber: 8.6g   Protein: 2g   Fat: 0.5g   Sugar: 38.5g

Minty Fresh

1 cup of chopped kale
½ cup of chopped parsley
3 mint leaves
1 cup of strawberry halves
1 cup of blueberries
1 cup of green tea

Directions:
Add the greens to the cup including the mint leaves. Follow with the berries and cooled green tea. Top up with filtered water if necessary. Blend until smooth.

Health Benefits
- Hydrates dry skin conditions.
- Reduces bad cholesterol levels.
- Reduces the risk of cancer.
- Provides relief from digestive discomfort.
- Decreases the risk of coronary heart disease.

Nutritional Information

Calories: 180   Dietary Fiber: 8.6g   Protein: 6.4g   Fat: 1.9g   Sugar: 22.3g

Precious Papaya

1 small papaya, cored
2 cups of spinach
1 cup of whole cranberries
1 teaspoon of matcha green tea powder
Filtered water

Directions:
Place the spinach into the cup first and follow with the papaya, cranberries, and matcha green tea powder. Add the filtered water and blend until smooth.

Health Benefits
- ❖ Aids weight loss by promoting a feeling of fullness.
- ❖ Strengthens the immune system.
- ❖ Helps to keep the eyes healthy.
- ❖ Protects against arthritis.
- ❖ Prevents signs of aging.

Nutritional Information

Calories: 142   **Dietary Fiber:** 10.2g   **Protein:** 2g   **Fat:** 0.7g   **Sugar:** 16.1g

Hail to Kale

2 cups of chopped kale
1 celery stalk, sliced
½ cucumber, sliced
2 kiwi fruit, peeled
1 cup of green tea

Directions:
Add the kale to the cup first and follow with the remaining ingredients. Pour in the cooled green tea and top up with filtered water if necessary.

Health Benefits
- Helps to manage blood pressure.
- Helps to eliminate toxins from the liver and blood.
- Prevents against constipation and other intestinal problems.
- Regulates the pH balance of blood.
- Promotes a good night's sleep.

Nutritional Information

Calories: 182   **Dietary Fiber:** 7.6g   **Protein:** 8.7g   **Fat:** 2.4g   **Sugar:** 15.2g

Pepper Pie

1 green pepper (sweet), seeded and chopped
1 cup of chopped asparagus
½ cup of blueberries
½ cup of pineapple chunks
1 cup of coconut water

Directions:
Place all prepared fruit and veg into the cup and add the coconut water. Top up with filtered water if necessary. Blend until smooth.

Health Benefits
- Promotes a feeling of fullness, helping with weight loss.
- Protects against colds and flu.
- Protects cells from free radical damage.
- Helps to promote wound healing.
- Delays the signs of aging.

Nutritional Information

Calories: 179 Dietary Fiber: 8.8g Protein: 5.1g Fat: 0.8g Sugar: 33.4g

Orange Supreme

2 carrots, peeled and sliced
1 orange, peeled and cut into segments
1 lime, peeled and cut into segments
½ teaspoon of turmeric
Filtered water

Directions:
Add all of the prepared ingredients into the cup and follow with the turmeric powder. Pour in the filtered water and blend until smooth.

Health Benefits
- Helps to reduce the risk of kidney disease and kidney stones.
- Boosts heart health.
- Fights against viral infection.
- Helps to regulate high blood pressure.
- Promotes healthy digestion.

Nutritional Information

Calories: 136   Dietary Fiber: 8.7g   Protein: 3.1g   Fat: 0.9g   Sugar: 19.1g

Green Delight

2 cups of watercress
1 cup of Swiss chard
½ avocado
1 wedge of lemon
1 level tablespoon of spirulina
1 cup of green tea

Directions:
Add the greens followed by the avocado, lemon, and spirulina. Pour in the cooled green tea and top up with filtered water if necessary. Blend until smooth.

Health Benefits
- Helps to reduce bad cholesterol.
- Promotes a healthy body weight and BMI.
- Helps to prevent the development of certain cancers.
- Improves skin tone and maintains good moisture levels in the skin.
- Helps to reduce arthritic pain.

Nutritional Information

Calories: 200   Dietary Fiber: 8.2g   Protein: 8.3g   Fat: 16.1g   Sugar: 7.8g

Magic Melon

1 cup of romaine lettuce, chopped
1 kiwi, peeled
1 cup of spinach
1 cup of watermelon chunks
1 cup of green tea
½ cup of crushed ice

Directions:
Place the leafy greens into the cup followed by the prepared fruit. Pour in the cooled green tea and top up with filtered water if necessary. Blend until smooth.

Health Benefits
- ❖ Lowers the risk of diabetes.
- ❖ Helps to build strong bones.
- ❖ Increases muscle strength.
- ❖ Helps to improve collagen synthesis.
- ❖ Improves cardiovascular health.

Nutritional Information

Calories: 105   Dietary Fiber: 4.4g   Protein: 3.2g   Fat: 0.8g   Sugar: 15.7g

Red River

1 cup of watercress
2 tomatoes, chopped
1 red pepper (sweet), seeded and chopped
1 carrot, peeled and sliced
1 level tablespoon of spirulina
1 cup of green tea

Directions:

Place the watercress into the cup and add the remaining prepared vegetables. Sprinkle the spirulina on top and pour in the cooled green tea. Top up with filtered water if necessary. Blend until smooth.

Health Benefits

- ❖ To promote the proper absorption of iron.
- ❖ Helps to reduce bloating.
- ❖ Helps to increase the metabolic rate of the body.
- ❖ Eases pre menstrual symptoms.
- ❖ Prevents against high blood pressure.

Nutritional Information

Calories: 132   Dietary Fiber: 6.9g   Protein: 9.6g   Fat: 1.6g   Sugar: 14.4g

Divine Nectarine

1 cup of red cabbage, chopped
1 cup of spinach
1 nectarine, cored
2 tangerines, peeled
Filtered water

Directions:
Add the red cabbage and spinach to the cup and follow with the nectarine and tangerines. Pour in the filtered water and blend until smooth.

Health Benefits
- Helps to relieve digestive disorders such as irritable bowel syndrome.
- Fights inflammation.
- Adds strength and support to muscles.
- Promotes collagen synthesis.
- Regulates bone mineralization.

Nutritional Information

Calories: 185   Dietary Fiber: 8.5g   Protein: 5.4g   Fat: 1g   Sugar: 31.9g

Gone Green

1 cup of collard greens
1 cup of chopped kale
1 cup of pineapple chunks
1 cup of strawberry halves
2 mint leaves
1 cup of green tea

Directions:
Add the leafy greens to the cup followed by the pineapple and strawberries. Pour in the cooled green tea and top up with filtered water if necessary. Blend until smooth.

Health Benefits
- ❖ Encourages smooth blood circulation.
- ❖ Lowers bad cholesterol levels.
- ❖ Helps to reduce the symptoms of osteoporosis.
- ❖ Reduces the risk of heart attack, stroke, and Alzheimer's disease.
- ❖ Helps to improve the firmness of our skin.

Nutritional Information

Calories: 177   Dietary Fiber: 7.7g   Protein: 5.9g   Fat: 1.5g   Sugar: 23.2g

<u>Glowing Green</u>

1 cup of green cabbage, shredded
½ cucumber, sliced
1 cup of bok choy, chopped
3 broccoli spears
2 wedges of lemon, peeled
1 cup of coconut water

Directions:
Place the leafy greens into the cup first and follow up with the remaining ingredients. Pour in the coconut water and top up with filtered water if necessary. Blend until smooth.

Health Benefits
- Helps to defends against colds and chest infections.
- Acts as a remedy for constipation.
- Reduces joint pain.
- Treats allergic reactions.
- Helps with weight loss by promoting a feeling of fullness.

Nutritional Information

Calories: 137   Dietary Fiber: 8.3g   Protein: 5.9g   Fat: 0.7g   Sugar: 20.3g

Banana Glory

1 cup of kale, chopped
1 peach, cored
1 banana, peeled and sliced
1 cup of green tea

Directions:
Add the kale to the cup first and follow with the banana and peach. Pour in the cooled green tea and top up with filtered water if necessary. Blend until smooth.

Health Benefits
- Helps to relieve urinary tract disorders.
- Builds strong bones.
- Enhances the body's metabolic rate.
- Protects against arthritis.
- Strengthens the immune system.

Nutritional Information

Calories: 199   Dietary Fiber: 6.3g   Protein: 5.6g   Fat: 1.4g   Sugar: 27g

Secret Sesame

2 cups of Swiss chard
1 cup of blackberries
1 small papaya, pitted
1 tablespoon of sesame seeds
Filtered water

Directions:
Add the Swiss chard followed by the blackberries, papaya, and sesame seeds. Pour in the filtered water and blend until smooth.

Health Benefits
- ❖ Helps to regulate bowel movement.
- ❖ Builds strong bones.
- ❖ Improves digestion.
- ❖ Boosts respiratory health.
- ❖ Helps to reduce type 2 diabetes.

Nutritional Information

Calories: 195 Dietary Fiber: 13g Protein: 5.5g Fat: 1.4g Sugar: 19.8g

Skinny Minnie

1 medium sized grapefruit, peeled
1 cup of diced watermelon
1 lime, peeled
1 passion fruit, without refuse
1 cup of green tea
½ cup of crushed ice

Directions:
Place all of the prepared fruit into the cup followed by the ice cubes and cooled green tea. Top up with filtered water if necessary and blend until smooth.

Health Benefits
- ❖ Provides relief from digestive disorders such as bloating and constipation.
- ❖ Promotes healthy gums and teeth.
- ❖ Protects against colds and flu.
- ❖ Increases the secretion of digestive enzymes, improving the digestion of food.
- ❖ Reduces the risk of heart disease.

Nutritional Information

Calories: 189   Dietary Fiber: 8.4g   Protein: 3.8g   Fat: 0.8g   Sugar: 28.1g

Gracious Grapes

2 cups of romaine lettuce
1 cup of red grapes
1 medium sized red pepper (sweet), seeded and chopped
1 beet, peeled and sliced
Filtered water

Directions:
Add the leafy greens to the cup followed by the grapes, red pepper, and beet. Sprinkle the matcha powder and pour in the filtered water. Blend until smooth.

Health Benefits
- ❖ Helps to relieve migraines.
- ❖ Boosts energy levels.
- ❖ Relieves constipation.
- ❖ Provides relief for indigestion and heartburn.
- ❖ Reduces the risk of a heart attack.

Nutritional Information

Calories: 192 **Dietary Fiber:** 7.3g **Protein:** 4.1g **Fat:** 0.6g **Sugar:** 35.2g

Liver Tonic

1 apple, cored
2 kiwi fruit, peeled
2 celery stalks, sliced
½ cup of crushed ice
Filtered water

Directions:
Place all of the prepared ingredients into the cup followed by the ice cubes. Pour in the filtered water and blend until smooth.

Health Benefits
- Relieves inflammation on problematic skin.
- Reduces acidity levels in the blood.
- Soothes the nervous system promoting peaceful sleep.
- Helps to cleanse the liver and blood.
- Protects against age related eye disorders.

Nutritional Information

Calories: 191   Dietary Fiber: 9.8g   Protein: 2.7g   Fat: 1.2g   Sugar: 32.4g

Veggie Heaven

1 green pepper (sweet), seeded and chopped
2 tomatoes, chopped
1 red pepper (sweet), seeded and chopped
1 small zucchini, sliced
1 cup of green tea

Directions:
Place all of the prepared ingredients into the cup and pour in the cooled green tea. Top up with filtered water if necessary and blend until smooth.

Health Benefits
- Helps to control diabetes.
- Eases the symptoms of allergic reactions.
- Healthy hair and skin.
- Provides relief from pain.
- Reduces the build up of bad cholesterol.

Nutritional Information

Calories: 140   Dietary Fiber: 9g   Protein: 6.6g   Fat: 1.2g   Sugar: 19.2g

Detox Deli

1 cup of red cabbage, chopped
1 cup of green cabbage, chopped
1 small papaya, cored
½ grapefruit, peeled
1 cup of green tea

Directions:
Add the red and green cabbage to the cup and follow with the papaya and grapefruit. Pour in the cooled green tea and top up with filtered water if necessary. Blend until smooth.

Health Benefits
- Strengthens weak, cracked fingernails.
- Reduces the symptoms of acne.
- Encourages better absorption of valuable nutrients.
- Helps to improve anemic conditions.
- Improves vision.

Nutritional Information

Calories: 165   **Dietary Fiber:** 9.1g   **Protein:** 3.9g   **Fat:** 0.8g   **Sugar:** 25.6g

Vitamin Frenzy

1 cup of strawberry halves
1 carrot, peeled and sliced
1 red pepper (sweet), seeded and sliced
10 almonds
1 teaspoon of matcha green tea powder
Filtered water

Directions:
Place all of the prepared ingredients into the cup. Add the almonds, matcha powder, and filtered water. Blend until smooth.

Health Benefits
- ❖ Helps to eliminate bad breath.
- ❖ Makes the body more alkaline.
- ❖ Revitalizes blood circulation in the lower legs.
- ❖ Soothes pain and inflammation.
- ❖ Speeds up the healing of wounds.

Nutritional Information

Calories: 196 **Dietary Fiber:** 9.2g **Protein:** 42.6g **Fat:** 10.7g **Sugar:** 14.9g

Cleanse & Detox

1 cucumber, sliced
2 celery stalks, sliced
1 beet, peeled and sliced
1" piece of ginger
1 cup of green tea

Directions:
Place all of the prepared fruit and veg into the cup along with the ginger. Pour in the green tea and top up with filtered water if necessary. Blend until smooth.

Health Benefits
- Helps to build muscle and improve exercise performance.
- Reduces sugar cravings in between meals.
- Improves mental clarity and focus.
- Relieves dry skin conditions such as dermatitis.
- Regulates bowel movements.

Nutritional Information

Calories: 105   Dietary Fiber: 5.4g   Protein: 4.1g   Fat: 0.7g   Sugar: 12.6g

Green Earth

½ cup of chopped parsley
1 cup of romaine lettuce, chopped
1 cup of watercress
1 cup of raspberries
2 plums, pitted
1 tablespoon of ground flax seeds
Filtered water

Directions:
Place the leafy greens into the cup first and follow with the fruit and flax seeds. Pour in the filtered water and blend until smooth.

Health Benefits
- ❖ Boosts metabolism and burns calories.
- ❖ Enhances moods and aids in concentration.
- ❖ Regulates blood sugar levels.
- ❖ Helps to fight against viruses and bacterial infections.
- ❖ Lowers bad cholesterol.

Nutritional Information

Calories: 185   Dietary Fiber: 13.9g   Protein: 6.1g   Fat: 7.6g   Sugar: 20g

Goji Crush

½ grapefruit, peeled and cut into segments
1 kiwi fruit, peeled
1 passion fruit, without the refuse
1 tablespoon of goji berries
½ cup of cranberries
½ cup of crushed ice
Filtered water

Directions:
Place all of the prepared fruit into the cup along with the crushed ice. Pour in the filtered water and blend until smooth.

Health Benefits
- Helps to fight gum disease.
- Protects against colds and flu.
- Reduces the risk of development cancer growths.
- Lowers acidic levels in the digestive system.
- Reduces the accumulation of fat deposits on arterial walls.

Nutritional Information

Calories: 176   Dietary Fiber: 10.4g   Protein: 4.4g   Fat: 1.1g   Sugar: 24g

Ocean Spring

1 cup of watercress
1 nectarine, pitted
1 orange, peeled and cut into segments
1 lime, peeled and cut into segments
1 tablespoon of ground flax seeds
1 cup of green tea

Directions:
Place the watercress into the cup first and follow with the prepared fruit and flax seeds. Pour in the cooled green tea and top up with filtered water if necessary. Blend until smooth.

Health Benefits
- Helps to promote sleep and alleviate insomnia.
- Reduces respiratory inflammation.
- Increases the flow of gastric juice in the stomach.
- Eases the symptoms of diabetes.
- Helps to absorb sugar in the body.

Nutritional Information

Calories: 187   Dietary Fiber: 9.5g   Protein: 5.8g   Fat: 3.5g   Sugar: 24.3g

Passionate Green

1 cup of spinach
1 cup of collard greens
1 passion fruit without the refuse
1 cup of mango pieces
1 cup of coconut water

Directions:
Add the leafy greens to the cup followed by the prepared fruit. Pour in the coconut water and top up with filtered water if necessary. Blend until smooth.

Health Benefits
- Reduces the risk of age-related diseases in the body.
- Enhances the absorption of iron in the intestines.
- Reduces the risk of cardiovascular disease, stroke, and heart attack.
- Helps to control digestive disorders such as diarrhea.
- Prevents against the formation of kidney stones.

Nutritional Information

Calories: 179   Dietary Fiber: 7.6g   Protein: 3.8g   Fat: 1g   Sugar: 37.8g

Green Attack

4 cauliflower flowerets
4 broccoli spears
1 cup of shredded boy choy
1 cup of chopped asparagus
Filtered water

Directions:
Place the boy choy into the cup first followed by the cauliflower, broccoli, and asparagus. Pour in the filtered water and blend until smooth.

Health Benefits
- ❖ Helps to treat skin irritations such as eczema.
- ❖ Stimulates venous circulation in the lower legs.
- ❖ Helps to reduce high blood pressure.
- ❖ Builds a strong immune system.
- ❖ Promotes healthy and strong muscles.

Nutritional Information

Calories: 92 **Dietary Fiber:** 7.9g **Protein:** 8.2g **Fat:** 0.7g **Sugar:** 5.9g

Fruit Punch

1 small papaya, pitted
1 cup of blackberries
½ cup of cherries without pits
1 cup of arugula
1 teaspoon of cinnamon
Filtered water

Directions:
Add the arugula to the cup first and follow with the blackberries, prepared papaya, and cherries. Sprinkle in the cinnamon and pour in the filtered water. Blend until smooth.

Health Benefits
- Helps to reduce inflammation in all forms of arthritis.
- Prevents constipation.
- Regulates the flow of menstruation in females.
- Reduces the symptoms of acne.
- Speeds up the elimination of toxins from the body.

Nutritional Information

Calories: 189   Dietary Fiber: 13.9g   Protein: 4.1g   Fat: 1.2g   Sugar: 29.3g

Antioxidant Apple

1 cup of watercress
1 apple, cored
1 orange, peeled and cut into segments
½ cup of whole cranberries
½ cup of crush ice
1 cup of green tea

Directions:
Add the watercress to the cup first and follow with the prepared fruit and crushed ice. Pour in the green tea and top up with filtered water if necessary. Blend until smooth.

Health Benefits
- ❖ Helps to treat stomach disorders such as peptic ulcers.
- ❖ Protects against viral and bacterial infections.
- ❖ Reduces the risk of heart disease.
- ❖ Fights free radical damage to reduce the risk of cancer.
- ❖ Stimulates digestion.

Nutritional Information

Calories: 186   Dietary Fiber: 10g   Protein: 1.9g   Fat: 0.7g   Sugar: 33.1g

Tangy Tank

1 cup of arugula
½ cup of chopped parsley
2 lemon wedges, peeled
1 cup of grapes
1 tablespoon of ground flax seed
Filtered water

Directions:
Add the arugula and parsley to the cup followed by the lemon and grapes. Sprinkle in the ground flax seed and pour in the filtered water. Blend until smooth.

Health Benefits
- Works at purifying the blood.
- Protects against inflammatory conditions such as arthritis.
- Helps to relieve bad breath.
- Reduces bloating and the build up of fluid.
- Healthy hair and nails.

Nutritional Information

Calories: 162   Dietary Fiber: 4.5g   Protein: 3.8g   Fat: 3.6g   Sugar: 23.9g

Ginger Banana

1 banana, peeled
2 cups of collard greens
½ cucumber, sliced
1" piece of ginger
1 level tablespoon of spirulina
Filtered water

Directions:
Place the collard greens into the cup and follow with the banana, cucumber and ginger. Sprinkle in the spirulina and pour in the filtered water. Blend until smooth.

Health Benefits
- ❖ Promotes brain function.
- ❖ Regulates the detoxification of the liver and blood.
- ❖ Improves skin's firmness and elasticity.
- ❖ Helps to burn fat cells at a faster rate.
- ❖ Improves vision and protects against age-related eye disorders.

Nutritional Information

Calories: 180   Dietary Fiber: 6.9g   Protein: 8.5g   Fat: 2.1g   Sugar: 17.1g

Orange & Lime

2 oranges, peeled and cut into segments
1 lime, peeled and cut into segments
½ cup of diced watermelon
½ cup of crushed ice
1 cup of green tea

Directions:

Add all of the prepared ingredients including the ice into the cup. Pour in the cooled green tea and top up with filtered water if necessary. Blend until smooth.

Health Benefits
- ❖ Improves bone health, repair, and development.
- ❖ Lowers bad cholesterol levels.
- ❖ Strengthens the immune system.
- ❖ Boosts the body's metabolism.
- ❖ Reduces anemia.

Nutritional Information

Calories: 169   Dietary Fiber: 8.4g   Protein: 3.8g   Fat: 0.6g   Sugar: 25.5g

Berry Star

1 cup of green cabbage, shredded
1 starfruit
1 cup of whole cranberries
1 cup of strawberry halves
1 tangerine, peeled
Filtered water

Directions:
Place the cabbage into the cup and add the starfruit, cranberries, strawberries, and tangerine. Pour in the filtered water and blend until smooth.

Health Benefits
- Has a gentle and cleansing effect on the digestive system.
- Speeds up wound healing.
- Prevents the development of certain cancers.
- Increases energy levels.
- Promotes regular bowel movements.

Nutritional Information

Calories: 192   Dietary Fiber: 13.9g   Protein: 4.2g   Fat: 1.3g   Sugar: 26.4g

Detox Splash

2 carrots, peeled and sliced
1 apple, cored
2 celery stalks, sliced
1 beet, peeled and sliced
1 cup of green tea

Directions:
Add all of the prepared fruit and veg into the cup. Pour in the cooled green tea and top up with filtered water if necessary. Blend until smooth.

Health Benefits
- ❖ Makes the body more alkaline.
- ❖ Eases congestion with respiratory disorders.
- ❖ Improves vision.
- ❖ Protects against free radical damage.
- ❖ Helps to fight against viral and bacterial infections.

Nutritional Information

Calories: 194   Dietary Fiber: 11.3g   Protein: 3.6g   Fat: 1g   Sugar: 32.2g

Summer Wave

1 cup of cherries, without pits
2 passion fruit, without refuse
1 cup of diced watermelon
1 teaspoon of cinnamon
½ cup of crushed ice
Filtered water

Directions:
Place the prepared fruit and ice into the cup and sprinkle in the cinnamon. Pour in the filtered water and blend until smooth.

Health Benefits
- ❖ Builds strong bones.
- ❖ Promotes healthy digestive function.
- ❖ Increases skin's ability to produce collagen.
- ❖ Helps to fight against bacterial infections in the stomach.
- ❖ Protects against age-related eye disorders.

Nutritional Information

Calories: 183   Dietary Fiber: 9g   Protein: 3.8g   Fat: 0.4g   Sugar: 33.1g

Green Blast

1 zucchini, sliced
½ cucumber, sliced
5 broccoli spears
1 tablespoon of pumpkin seeds
1 level tablespoon of spirulina
1 cup of green tea

Directions:
Place the prepared veg into the cup, add the pumpkin seeds, and sprinkle in the spirulina. Pour in the cooled green tea and top up with filtered water if necessary. Blend until smooth.

Health Benefits
- Protects against inflammation in the respiratory tract.
- Regulates blood glucose levels.
- Improves digestive function.
- Helps with the formation and development of cells.
- Reduces dandruff and helps to prevent against hair loss.

Nutritional Information

Calories: 194   Dietary Fiber: 7.3g   Protein: 11.9g   Fat: 7.2g   Sugar: 9.9g

Fruitilicious

1 banana, peeled and sliced
2 cups of diced watermelon
Filtered water

Directions:
Add the prepared banana and watermelon into the cup. Pour in the filtered water and blend until smooth.

Health Benefits
- Increases energy levels.
- Improves brain function.
- Relieves indigestion and heartburn.
- Promotes muscular health.
- Eases the feelings of stress.

Nutritional Information

Calories: 197   Dietary Fiber: 4.3g   Protein: 3.1g   Fat: 0.8g   Sugar: 32g

Nutrient Ninja

1 cup of spinach
1 cup of raspberries
1 cup of grapes
1 tomato, sliced
Filtered water

Directions:
Add the spinach to the cup first and follow with the fruit and tomato. Pour in the filtered water and blend until smooth.

Health Benefits
- ❖ Helps to reduce the growth and development of cancer cells.
- ❖ Promotes a feeling of fullness, helping with weight loss.
- ❖ Reduces age spots and discolorations on the skin.
- ❖ Protects against bacterial infections such as colds.
- ❖ Strengthens connective tissue.

Nutritional Information

Calories: 198   Dietary Fiber: 11.2g   Protein: 4.1g   Fat: 1.4g   Sugar: 31.3g

Berry Rejuvenator

2 cups of strawberry halves
1 tablespoon of goji berries
1 cup of Swiss chard
1 cup of coconut water

Directions:
Place the Swiss chard into the cup first and follow with the strawberries and goji berries. Pour in the coconut water and top up with filtered water if necessary. Blend until smooth.

Health Benefits
- ❖ Provides relief from arthritis and gout.
- ❖ Reduces the signs of premature aging.
- ❖ Strengthens the immune system.
- ❖ Reduces the risk of eye related disorders.
- ❖ Enhances memory concentration.

Nutritional Information

Calories: 192   Dietary Fiber: 10.3g   Protein: 4.6g   Fat: 1.4g   Sugar: 32.9g

Leafy Green

1 cup of watercress
1 cup of collard greens, chopped
1 cup of kale, chopped
2 kiwi fruit, peeled
2 wedges of lemon, peeled
1 cup of green tea

Directions:
Add the leafy greens to the cup first followed by the kiwi fruit and lemon. Pour in the green tea and top up with filtered water if necessary. Blend until smooth.

Health Benefits
- Promotes the healthy function of the digestive system.
- Protects the cells against free radical damage.
- Helps with the absorption of iron in the blood.
- Balances the body's fluids.
- Regulates blood pressure.

Nutritional Information

Calories: 138   Dietary Fiber: 5.1g   Protein: 6.6g   Fat: 1.6g   Sugar: 17.2g

Amazing Asparagus

1 cup of whole cranberries
1 cup of blackberries
1 cup of chopped asparagus
1 tablespoon of ground flax seed
1 level tablespoon of spirulina
1 cup of green tea

Directions:
Add the berries, asparagus, and flax seed, sprinkle in the spirulina, and pour in the cooled green tea. Top up with filtered water if necessary and blend until smooth.

Health Benefits
- ❖ Promotes younger looking skin.
- ❖ Balances the internal pH of the body.
- ❖ Alleviates low moods.
- ❖ Promotes a good night's sleep.
- ❖ Helps to lower bad cholesterol levels.

Nutritional Information

Calories: 194 Dietary Fiber: 17.3g Protein: 10.7g Fat: 5g Sugar: 13.6g

The Green King

1 cup of chopped kale
1 cup of arugula
2 lemon wedges, peeled
1 cucumber, sliced
1 cup of coconut water

Directions:
Add the leafy greens followed by the lemon and cucumber. Pour in the coconut water and blend until smooth.

Health Benefits
- ❖ Reduces the risk of cancer.
- ❖ Reduces the symptoms of osteoporosis.
- ❖ Improves brain function.
- ❖ Boosts the body's metabolic rate.
- ❖ Decreases the risk of chronic disease.

Nutritional Information

Calories: 135   Dietary Fiber: 3.9g   Protein: 5.4g   Fat: 1g   Sugar: 18.1g

Orange Infusion

1 cup of romaine lettuce, chopped
2 tangerines, peeled
2 carrots, peeled and sliced
1 green pepper (sweet), seeded and chopped
½ cup of crushed ice
Filtered water

Directions:
Add the romaine lettuce to the cup first and follow with the prepared fruit and veg. Add the crushed ice, pour in the filtered water, and blend until smooth.

Health Benefits
- Aids weight loss by creating a feeling of fullness.
- Increases energy levels and stamina.
- Helps to balance the pH of the blood.
- Helps to improve collagen production in the skin.
- Reduces the build up of bad cholesterol in the arteries.

Nutritional Information

Calories: 176   Dietary Fiber: 9.6g   Protein: 4.2g   Fat: 1.3g   Sugar: 27.3g

References

Jonny Bowden, Ph,D., C.N.S., *The 150 Healthiest Foods on Earth.* Fair Winds Press, 2007.

Nutrient Data for ingredients listed was provided by USDA. *http://ndb.nal.usda.gov/ndb/foods*

Nutribullet LLC, *Nutribullet User Guide & Recipe Book.*

Paul Pitchford, *Healing with Whole Foods Asian Traditions and Modern Nutrition,* North Atlantic Books, U.S., 2002.

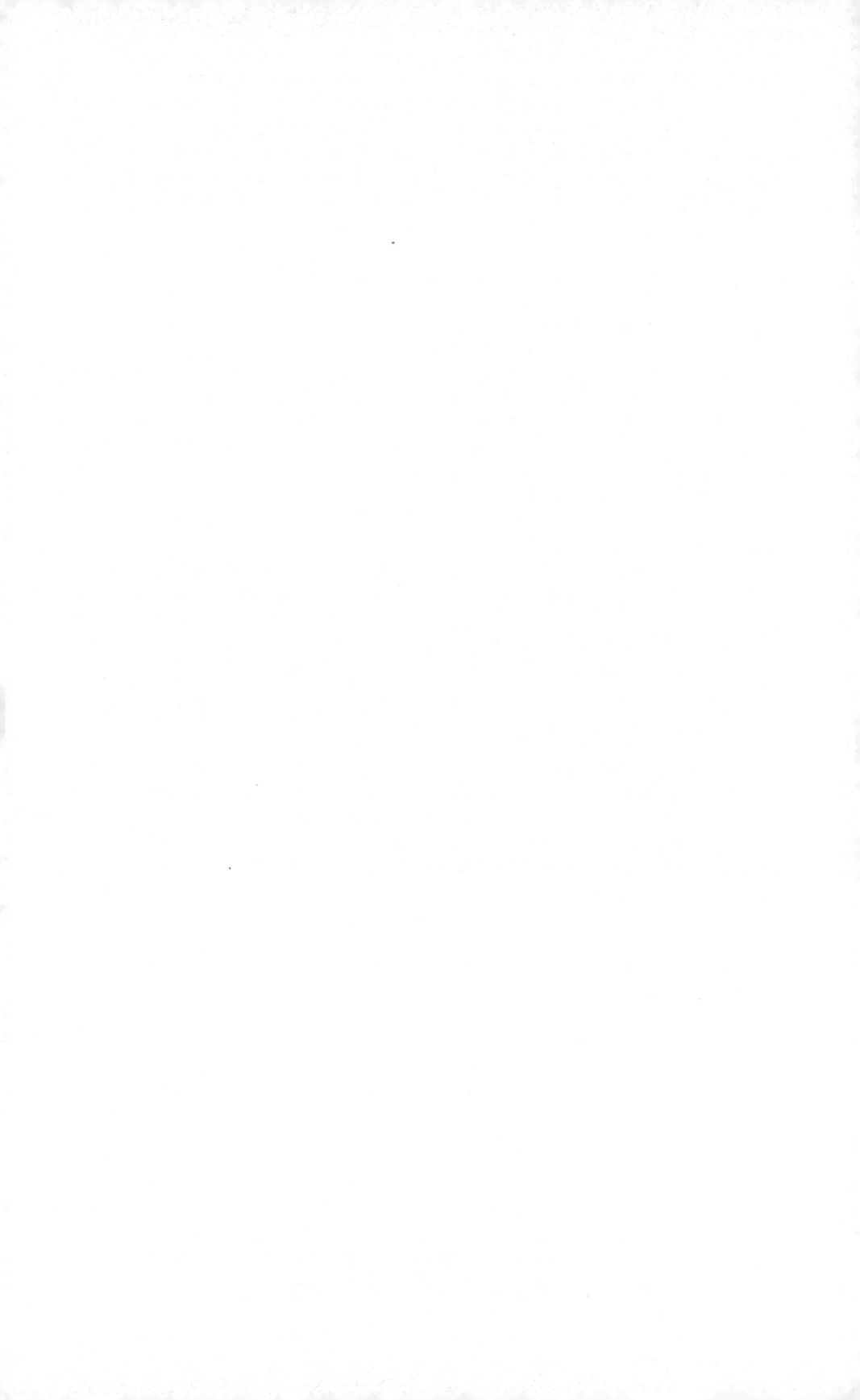

Printed in Great Britain
by Amazon